Clean Eating

Irresistible Clean Eating Recipes for Effortless Weight Loss and Vibrant Health

By Cassia Albinson

Copyright © Cassia Albinson 2016

All rights reserved. No part of this publication may be reproduced, stored in a retrieval system, or transmitted, in any form or by any means, electronic, mechanical, photocopying, recording or otherwise, without the prior written permission of the author and the publishers.

Cassia Albinson © Copyright 2016 - All rights reserved.

Legal Notice:

This book is copyright protected. It for personal use only. You cannot amend, distribute, sell, use, quote or paraphrase any part or the content within this book without the consent of the author or copyright owner. Legal action will be pursued if this is breached.

Disclaimer Notice:

Please note the information contained in this document is for educational and entertainment purposes only. Every attempt has been made to provide accurate, up to date and completely reliable information. No warranties of any kind are expressed or implied.

Readers acknowledge that the author is not engaging in the rendering of legal, financial, medical or professional advice. By reading this document, the reader agrees that under no circumstances are we responsible for any losses, direct or indirect, which are incurred as a result of the use of information contained within this document, including, but not limited to, errors, omissions, or inaccuracies.

Contents

Clean Eating Introduction 6

Free eBook 9

Breakfasts 11

    Protein Pancake 12

    Peanut Butter Apple Cinnamon Bran Muffins 16

    Peanut Butter Apple Cinnamon Bran Muffin French Toast 21

    Organic Apple Oatmeal Cooked in Cinnamon Rooibos Infusion 23

    Organic Coffee, Coconut and Tahini Oat Bran 25

    Banana Peanut Butter Protein Smoothie 27

    Berrylicious Smoothie 29

    Overnight Oatmeal Energy Bowl 31

    Egg in the Hole 33

    Apple Treat 36

    Banana Bread Breakfast Cookies 38

Lunches 40

    Sundried Tomato and Black Olive Frittata 41

    Lentil and Veggie Packed Omelet 43

    Zucchini Taco Boats 46

    Veggie Burgers with Avocado 49

    Soba Noodles with Sesame, Kale, and Brussels Sprouts 51

Roast Butternut and Goat's Cheese Frittata 54

Fresh Hake or Cod Cakes 57

Roast Butternut Salad with Organic Free Range Hard Boiled Eggs 59

Chick Pea, Goat's Cheese and Organic Greens Salad 61

Organic Free Range Egg Omelette with Goat's Cheese and Free Range Smoked Trout 63

Quinoa Salad with Seared Free-Range Tuna 65

Healthy Snacks 68

Organic Granny Smith Apple Slices with Fresh Ginger and Chopped Pecan Nuts 69

Organic Red Apple Slices with Organic Peanut Butter and Dried Cranberries 71

Organic Goat's Cheese with Fresh Organic Crudités 73

Fresh Organic Berries with Organic Goat's Milk Yogurt and Raw Almonds 75

Fresh Organic Avocado Guacamole with Fresh Organic Crudités 77

Dinners 79

Fresh Free Range Salmon Curry with Coconut Milk, Roast Butternut and Brown Rice 81

Baked Fresh Free Range Hake or Cod with Roast Vegetables and Quinoa 83

Whole Wheat Pasta Bake with Roast Vegetables, Black Olives and Goat's Milk Cheese 86

Roast Vegetable and Black Olive Patties 88

Vegetarian Chili with Brown Rice and Black Olives 90

Fresh Whole Free Range Trout with Fresh Organic Greens 92

Vegetarian Lasagne with Organic Goat's Cheese Topping 94

Chick Pea and Sweet Potato Curry with Quinoa 96

Chicken with Brussels Sprouts and Mustard Sauce 98

Lemony Chicken Kebabs with Tomato Salad 101

Mediterranean Stuffed Chicken Breasts 104

Shrimp and Avocado Rolls 106

Thai Chopped Salad with Curry Coconut Dressing 109

Goodbye and Good Natural Health 112

Free Complimentary eBook .... **Error! Bookmark not defined.**

More Books Written by Cassia 115

Clean Eating Introduction

Once you become aware of the benefits of clean eating you'll wonder why had never taken on such a lifestyle before; and you will never look back. In recent years there has been a steady growth in the worldwide awareness to the necessity of knowing exactly what you are eating, and in taking complete control of it. Not only is this approach the best for your overall health, but it is also the safest and most nutritious way to achieve and maintain a healthy weight, sustained energy and a strong immune system.

By taking on the clean eating approach you are eliminating many of the toxins that come in the form of preservatives, additives, artificial flavours and stabilisers that are common ingredients in processed and pre-packaged foods. Many of these additives have been known to cause a number of types of cancers, and the high sugar content of so many processed and pre-packaged foods can lead to Type 2 diabetes. The high fat content of many of these processed and pre-packaged foods can lead to high cholesterol and heart disease.

By choosing to take complete, or as much control as is possible over what you eat and how your meals are prepared, you can be assured that you are feeding your body holistically and at the same time preventing lifestyle induced illnesses.

Organic fresh produce provides you with the richest sources of vitamins and minerals and is free of disease and allergy causing pesticides; not to mention how buying from your local organic farmer's market will reduce the amount of packaging required and therefore is kinder to the environment.

Organic free range eggs are always the best choice and will always provide you with the peace of mind that you are not exposing yourself to any potential diseases or bacteria that may have penetrated the porous shell; also, free range organically farmed hens are of the healthiest and eat natural wholegrain diets, ensuring that the eggs they produce are of top quality.

The choice of freshly caught fish is not only kinder to the environment but is also a way of ensuring that you are eating a top quality protein source that is free of any anti-biotics or contamination from the water in which farmed fish will come from.

Cheeses and yogurts made from organic goat's milk is a very healthy source of calcium as well as essential amino acids and minerals. By choosing organic "dairy" products such as this you are eliminating the risk of ingesting any hormones or anti-biotics that are widely used in cattle dairy farming.

With all the organic, clean food options available to you there is no reason why you can't take control of your eating and lifestyle. This book aims to provide you with hearty, healthy and wholesome recipes that will inspire you to live life the healthy way and to feed your body only the very best of ingredients at every meal time.

Free eBook + Free Wellness Newsletter

Before we dive into it…We have a free, complimentary eBook for you.

It's waiting for you at:

www.YourWellnessBooks.com/newsletter

Problems with your download?

Email us at: info@yourwellnessbooks.com

Breakfasts

When making the decision to start living a healthy, lifestyle the first thing one needs to do is to start having breakfast *every day!* Breakfast really is the most important meal of the day because it breaks the fast of sleeping and kick starts your metabolism for the day; which is essential for weight loss and weight maintenance. The problem with many convenience breakfasts such as ready-made processed cereals, is that they are high in sugar and unhealthy fats; many of them also have a high glyceamic index, which means that they spike your blood sugar levels and then drop them rapidly, leaving you ravenous an hour later. A healthy, wholesome and nutritious breakfast that includes a good balance of slow releasing carbohydrates, protein and healthy fats is the best way to start your day and to stabilise blood sugar levels from the start. The recipes in this section are all easy to prepare and will promise to give you everything thing you need to start every day in a healthy way.

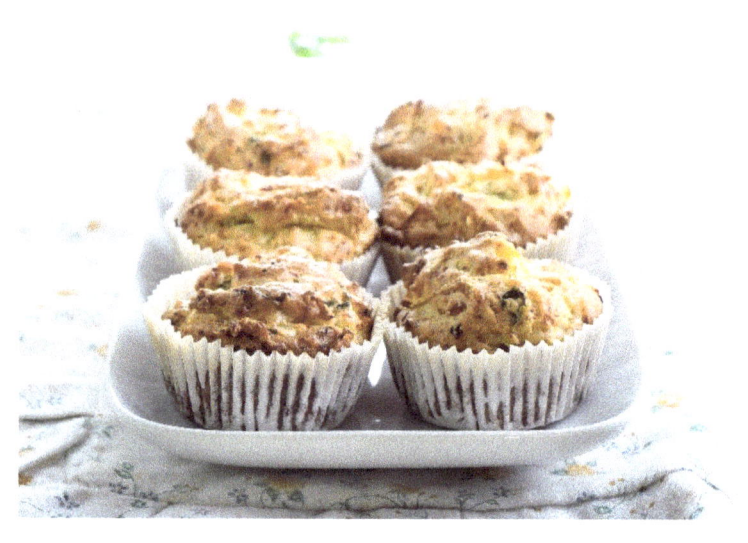

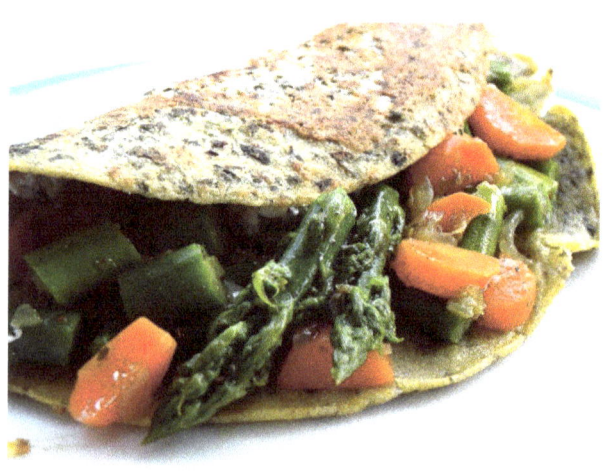

Protein Pancake

As mentioned in the introduction to this book; organic free range eggs are an amazing protein source. An egg could essentially be labelled as a whole meal on its own since it contains a good balance of protein, essential amino acids, vitamins, minerals, omega 3s and healthy fats. Over the last few years eggs have gotten a bad name amongst health enthusiasts due to their cholesterol content, but many studies have proven this line of thought to be completely incorrect. In fact, studies have shown that eggs contain healthy amounts of cholesterol and can be included in your diet to help lower your cholesterol and maintain a healthy level. It's all about how you cook your eggs and your overall lifestyle that makes the difference. This recipe will provide you with a well-balanced breakfast that will definitely not leave you racing for the vending machine as soon as you arrive at work.

Serves One

Preparation time: approximately 20 minutes

Ingredients:

- 1 large organic free range egg
- ¼ teaspoon (1.25ml) Ground Cinnamon
- ¼ teaspoon (1.25ml) Raw Cocoa Powder

- ¼ teaspoon (1.25ml) Vanilla essence
- ¼ teaspoon (1.25ml) Baking powder
- 1 Tablespoon (15ml) Almond milk

Instructions:

1. Lightly spray a non-stick frying pan with non-stick spray and place on the stove top on a medium heat
2. Place all the ingredients into a mixing bowl and whisk until light and fluffy
3. Pour the ingredients into the pan and allow to cook slowly; when the pancake is ready to be turned over it will start lifting off the base of the pan on its own
4. Once the pancake is cooked, turn it out onto a dinner plate and fill it with one of the following options:

Filling option 1:

Ingredients:

- 1 medium sized banana
- 1 teaspoon (5ml) organic sugar-free fruit preserve
- 1 Tablespoon (15m) Chopped raw nuts of your choice (eg, walnuts, almonds, cashews or pecans)

Instructions:

1. Spread the fruit preserve over the entire surface area of the pancake
2. Slice the banana and place it along the edge of one side of the pancake
3. Sprinkle the chopped nuts over the banana
4. Roll up the pancake and enjoy

Filling option 2 (this is a great option if you are packing your pancake to go):

Ingredients:

- 1 teaspoon (5ml) Organic peanut butter (any nut butter will do really, it's your choice)
- 1 teaspoon (5ml) organic sugar-free fruit preserve

Instructions:

1. Spread the peanut butter over the entire surface area of the pancake
2. Spread the organic fruit preserve over the peanut butter
3. Roll up the pancake and enjoy.

Peanut Butter Apple Cinnamon Bran Muffins

Wholegrain carbohydrates are a wonderful source of slow releasing energy and are a great way to stabilise and maintain blood sugar levels. Carbohydrates are necessary for the body to function correctly, particularly the brain; when you chose to consume the right kinds of carbohydrates in sufficient serving sizes then there is no reason to give them a bad name as many new fad diets do. The inclusion of cinnamon in this recipe not only gives it that comforting flavour, but also brings along all the health benefits of cinnamon, which include anti-inflammatory as well as blood sugar regulating properties. You will also notice that this recipe does not include sugar; when you taste the result you will see how it is not necessary to bake with refined sugar and that the apple provides sufficient sweetness the healthy way. These muffins are quick and easy to whip up, can be made in advance, are suitable for home freezing, and can be eaten as part of a breakfast or as a snack, as you will see with the recipes to follow this one.

Makes 30 muffins

Preparation time; approximately 45 minutes

Ingredients:

- 1 ¼ Cup (300grams) Organic whole wheat flour
- ¼ Cup (60ml) Organic wheat bran

- 2 teaspoons (10ml) baking powder
- 1 tablespoon (15ml) Ground cinnamon
- 1 tablespoon (15ml) Raw cocoa powder
- 1 tablespoon (15ml) Organic smooth peanut butter
- 1 large red apple, cored and grated (it is recommended that you don't peel the apple so to keep the extra fibre and nutrients found in the skin)
- 2 eggs
- 1 Cup (250ml) Almond milk
- 1 ½ Cups (375ml) Cinnamon infused Rooibos tea infusion (see below)
- 1 Tablespoon (15ml) Vanilla essence
- ½ Cup (125ml) Organic goat's milk yogurt (you can also use coconut yoghurt)

For the Cinnamon infused Rooibos tea:

Either plain or fruit flavoured Rooibos tea can be used. This infusion is made in a tea pot with an infusion basket and allowed to steep over night.

To make the Rooibos infusion:

1. Fill the infusion basket of your teapot half way, with organic cinnamon sticks or bark.
2. Place two Rooibos tea bags on top of the cinnamon. If you are using loose tea leaves, you will need approximately four teaspoons (20ml) of the leaves.
3. Fill the pot with boiling water, and allow to steep overnight.

Instructions to make the muffins:

Preheat the oven to 375 degrees (200 degrees Celsius)

Spray two and half small muffin trays with non-stick spray

1. Place the whole wheat flour, wheat bran, baking powder, ground cinnamon, raw cocoa powder and grated apple into a large mixing bowl and combine.
2. Crack the eggs into a separate mixing bowl and add the almond milk, goat's milk yogurt, Rooibos tea infusion and the peanut butter. Whisk together until all combined, light and fluffy
3. Add the wet ingredients to the dry and mix thoroughly; making sure that everything is well combined.

4. Using a 1 Tablespoon (15ml) measuring spoon, spoon the muffin mix into the muffin trays placing 1 tablespoon (15ml) of the muffin mix into each cavity at a time.

5. Once you have placed 1 tablespoon (15ml) of the muffin mix into each cavity of the muffin trays, repeat step 4 until all the muffin mix is in the muffin trays. By doing this you are ensuring that each muffin has an equal quantity of muffin mix to it.

6. Bake for 25 minutes.

7. Once baked allow to cool in the muffin tins for about 10 minutes before turning out onto a cooling rack.

To Serve:

These muffins are light and fluffy and go very well with any topping you may desire; here are some examples:

- Organic peanut butter
- Organic sugar-free fruit preserve
- Organic goat's milk cheese
- Fresh banana
- Poached organic free range eggs

- Organic goat's milk yogurt or coconut yoghurt

Peanut Butter Apple Cinnamon Bran Muffin French Toast

French toast is a childhood favourite for many and is usually made using stale white bread that has been soaked in beaten eggs and then fried in a frying pan. This recipe uses the previous muffin recipe as a fresh, much healthier take on the classic recipe. This breakfast will provide you with a tasty balance of healthy carbohydrate, protein and fat that you don't have to feel guilty about at all; just another way to see how you can treat yourself in a healthy way.

Serves One

Preparation time: Approximately 15-20 minutes

Ingredients:

- Two Peanut Butter Apple Cinnamon Bran Muffins
- 1 large organic free range egg
- 1 Tablespoon (15ml) Almond milk

Instructions:

1. Spray a non-stick pan with cooking spray and place on the stove top at a medium heat
2. In a flat dish (a pie dish will work perfectly) whisk the egg and almond milk together

3. Slice the muffins in half and place them in the egg and almond milk mixture

4. Allow the muffins to sit in the egg mixture for a few minutes, turning over every now and then, until they have absorbed all of the egg mixture.

5. Once the muffins have absorbed all of the egg mixture, place them in the now warm frying pan and cook on either side until golden brown.

6. Serve hot with one or more of the following topping options:

- Organic peanut butter

- Organic sugar-free fruit preserve

- Organic goat's milk cheese

- Fresh banana (or any fruit)

- Organic goat's milk yogurt

Organic Apple Oatmeal Cooked in Cinnamon Rooibos Infusion

This recipe brings a new and interesting way to cooking good old traditional oatmeal, it is quick and easy to prepare and provides you with a very wholesome energy rich breakfast that will definitely start your day off on a high note. This recipe also provides a great breakfast option for straight after a really hard morning exercise session. This recipe is cooked in the microwave for convenience sake, however can be done on the stove top should you prefer not to use a microwave; note that cooking on the stove top will add at least another ten minutes to the preparation time.

Serves one

Preparation time: approximately 15 minutes

Ingredients:

- ¼ Cup (60ml) Raw Organic quick cooking oats
- 1 small apple, cored and grated (it is recommended that you don't peel the apple so as to keep all the nutrients that are found in the skin)
- 1 Tablespoon (15ml) Raw seed mix
- ½ Cup (250ml) Cinnamon Rooibos infusion (see above)
- ¼ teaspoon (1.25ml) Ground cinnamon

- 1 teaspoon (5ml) Raw cocoa powder
- ½ Cup (250ml) almond milk (for serving)
- 1 teaspoon (5ml) Organic peanut butter (for serving)

Instructions:

1. Place the cinnamon infused rooibos tea in a microwavable cup or jug and heat on high for about 1 minute (you want to get it up to boiling point)
2. Place the oats, grated apple, raw seed mix, raw cocoa powder and ground cinnamon in a microwavable bowl, mix together
3. Add the now hot cinnamon rooibos tea infusion, stir together well
4. Cook in the microwave for two minutes on high
5. Once the oats are cooked, stir in the peanut butter
6. Place the almond milk in a microwaveable cup or jug and heat on a medium-low heat in the microwave
7. Add the now warm almond milk to your oats, stir well and enjoy.

Organic Coffee, Coconut and Tahini Oat Bran

We all love our morning cup of coffee, and there is absolutely no reason that we can't enjoy it while still leading a healthy lifestyle. Many studies have shown that pure organic coffee has loads of health benefits; it is high in anti-oxidants, great for asthma sufferers, can help lower blood pressure, and boosts serotonin. This recipe provides you with a very tasty breakfast option that is not only wholesome and healthy, but also fresh and exciting; it is also another great breakfast option after a hard morning exercise session. This recipe is also cooked in the microwave, but can be done on the stove top if preferred; just add another 10 minutes to your cooking time.

Serves one

Preparation time: approximately 15 minutes

Ingredients:

- ¼ Cup (60ml) Raw Organic oat bran
- 1 Tablespoon (15ml) Desiccated coconut
- 1 teaspoon (5ml) Raw cocoa powder
- ¼ teaspoon (2.5ml) Ground cinnamon
- ½ Cup (250ml) Organic filter coffee (at boiling point)

- 1 teaspoon (5ml) Tahini (for serving)
- 1 small banana (for serving)
- ¼ Cup (60ml) almond milk (for serving)

Instructions:

1. Place the oat bran, desiccated coconut, raw cocoa powder and ground cinnamon into a microwaveable bowl, mix together
2. Add the hot filter coffee
3. Cook in the microwave on a high setting for 2 minutes
4. Once the oat bran is cooked, stir in the Tahini
5. Slice the banana into the oat bran
6. Place the almond milk into a microwaveable cup or jug and heat on a medium-low heat for 1 minute
7. Add the now warm almond milk to the oat bran and mix well before tucking in to enjoy.

Banana Peanut Butter Protein Smoothie

Smoothies are great quick and easy way to get a nutritious well-balanced breakfast in. This recipe combines the healthy carbohydrate and potassium richness of bananas with the healthy fats provided by the peanut butter. By adding raw oats to the mixture we are amping up the fibre content, as well as adding more energy sustaining bulk. The addition of the raw egg gives you all the nutrient value of the egg in its entirety without any loss caused by the cooking process. The raw cocoa powder adds extra anti-oxidants and amino acids to the combination, as well as a rich chocolaty flavour. This smoothie can be made advance and kept in the refrigerator if necessary.

Serves one:

Preparation time: approximately 10 minutes

Ingredients:

- 1 large banana
- ¼ cup (60ml) Raw organic oats
- 1 Cup (250ml) Organic goat's milk yogurt
- 1 Cup (250ml) Cinnamon Rooibos tea infusion
- 1 Tablespoon (15ml) Organic peanut butter

- 1 large organic free range egg, raw
- 1 teaspoon (5ml) Raw cocoa powder

Instructions:

1. Slice the banana into the jug of a blender
2. Add the goat's milk yogurt, cinnamon rooibos tea, peanut butter, raw egg and cocoa powder
3. Blend until smooth and enjoy, serve chilled

Berrylicious Smoothie

This recipe gives another example of a healthy breakfast smoothie; the berries bring along essential antioxidants and high vitamin C content, while the raw oats provides extra fibre. This smoothie also includes a raw egg as the protein portion of this smoothie.

Serves one:

Preparation time: approximately 10 minutes

Ingredients:

- 1 Cup (250ml) mixed fresh or frozen berries (this can include raspberries, gooseberries, strawberries, blue berries and black berries; your choice really)

- 1 Cup (250ml) Organic goat's milk yogurt

- 1 Cup (250ml) Cinnamon Rooibos tea infusion

- 1 teaspoon (5ml) Raw cocoa powder

- 1 Tablespoon (15ml) Desiccated coconut

- ¼ Cup (60ml) Raw organic oats

- 1 large organic free range egg, raw *(optional), you can use hemp or some plant based protein powder instead*

Instructions:

1. Place all the ingredients into the jug of a blender and blend until smooth

2. Serve chilled

Overnight Oatmeal Energy Bowl

Oatmeal is one of the best energy based foods you can have for breakfast. It is even better when you add to the favorite hot cereal with protein and fruit. Not only do you gain fiber in your diet, but you also gain more nutrients depending on the garnishes you add to your oatmeal energy bowl. All it takes is ten minutes of prep to truly have a great dish for breakfast, so it is not like you have to forgo the most important meal of the morning, either. To make this the cleanest recipe for weight loss ensure you are using gluten free oats.

SERVES: One

PREPARATION TIME: 10 minutes

INGREDIENTS:

- 1 ripe banana
- 2 tablespoons (30 ml) Chia seeds
- ¼ teaspoon (1.42 grams) cinnamon
- 1/3 cup (76 grams) oats
- 2/3 cup (157 ml) almond milk
- 1 tablespoon (15 ml) ground flax seed
- 1 handful almonds or other nuts

INSTRUCTIONS:

1. In a medium bowl, mash a banana until smooth.
2. Add in all ingredients, except the almonds or nuts of your choice.
3. Cover and place in the fridge overnight.
4. Scoop the oatmeal into a pot in the morning.
5. Bring the mixture to a boil.
6. Reduce heat to medium, and simmer for five minutes.
7. Pour oatmeal mixture into a bowl.
8. Garnish with the nuts

ADDITIONAL SUGGESTIONS:

The prep time at night will help rolled oats become softer. You can use a different type of gluten free oats that will not take an overnight preparation. You can also garnish with a little toasted coconut, nut butter, or allspice depending on your tastes.

Egg in the Hole

Squash and range, free chicken eggs make a great clean recipe for breakfast. You gain protein from the eggs, as well as dress them up with some healthy anti-oxidants, vitamins, and additional protein. Since you are not eating this, every day, you will not have to worry about the cholesterol of the eggs. The cholesterol is also lowered by how you cook the eggs.

SERVES: One to Six

PREPARATION TIME: Approximately 40 minutes

INGREDIENTS:

- 6 whole, range free eggs
- 2 acorn squash
- 5 pitted dates
- 2 tablespoons (30 ml) coconut oil
- 8 walnut halves
- Parsley for garnish

INSTRUCTIONS:

1. Prcheat your oven to 375 degrees F (190 degrees C).

2. Slice the squash crosswise to get at least 3 slices out of each squash. You should make the slices about ¾ inch thick.

3. Remove the seeds from the center of the squash slices.

4. Place the squash slices on a baking sheet.

5. Sprinkle with a light touch of salt and pepper.

6. Bake for 20 minutes.

7. Using a nut chopper or food processor, chop the nuts and dates to get a texture that is similar to coarse sand.

8. When the timer beeps, remove the squash from the oven.

9. Drizzle the coconut oil evenly over each slice.

10. Crack an egg directly into the center of each squash slice.

11. Add the date/walnut crumble to the top of the egg and squash slices.

12. Return the baking sheet to the oven with your squash doctored slices, for 10 minutes or until the eggs are done to your liking.

13. Remove from the oven.

14. Garnish the slices with parsley, if you wish.

15. Serve.

ADDITIONAL SUGGESTIONS:

You can make this to serve one by reducing the slices you bake and the eggs you use. You can also add a hint of maple syrup, again a sugar free, gluten free concoction for healthy, clean eating, to help dress up the egg in the hole.

Apple Treat

Apples are healthy and meant to provide your body with anti-oxidants, immunity properties, and vitamins that are essential for living a clean, healthy life. Apples can also help with weight loss given their low calorie amount.

SERVES: One

PREPARATION TIME: Approximately 6 minutes

INGREDIENTS:

- 1 tablespoon (15 ml) organic butter or coconut oil
- 2 tablespoons (15 ml) applesauce
- ¼ teaspoon (1.42 grams) vanilla
- 1 free range chicken egg
- 3 tablespoons (45 ml) almond flour
- 1 teaspoon (5.69 grams) maple syrup
- ½ teaspoon (2.84 grams) cinnamon
- 1/8 teaspoon (0.7 grams) baking powder
- 1 tablespoon (15 ml) apple, chopped finely
- A pinch of chopped walnuts

INSTRUCTIONS:

1. Melt the butter in your microwave safe mug.

2. Whisk in the applesauce, egg, maple syrup, and vanilla.

3. Add the almond flour, baking powder, cinnamon, and stir for 30 seconds.

4. Add in the apples and walnuts on the top.

5. Microwave for 1 minute and 10 seconds.

6. Let the mug cool for a few minutes.

ADDITIONAL SUGGESTIONS:

If you wish, you can add to this recipe to increase the servings. To bake the muffins, turn the oven on to 350 degrees F (176 degrees C), melt the butter in the microwave and then follow the mixing steps as above. You can either place it in a baking dish or use a mug for each serving. If you bake the muffin mixture you will need to keep them in the oven for 25 minutes.

Banana Bread Breakfast Cookies

Banana Bread Breakfast Cookies are perfect for anyone looking to have a dairy free, gluten free meal. You can make this vegan, vegetarian, and nut free if you wish. The oatmeal and cranberries are two perfect ingredients for fiber and dietary regulation. Both are known to help with any digestive issues you might have.

SERVES: Six

PREPARATION TIME: Approximately 15 minutes

INGREDIENTS:

- 2 cups gluten free oats
- 2 large bananas
- ½ cup (113 grams) dried cranberries

INSTRUCTIONS:

1. Preheat oven to 350 degrees F (176 degrees C)
2. Using a food processor, blend the oats until it becomes a flour consistency.
3. In a large bowl, mash the banana until smooth.
4. Mix in the oats, until they are well mixed with the bananas.
5. Add in the cranberries.

6. Spray a cookie sheet with a gluten free, clean cooking spray or butter.

7. Drop the oatmeal dough on the cookie sheet, about a tablespoon per drop.

8. Flatten the dough with a rubber, non-stick spatula.

9. Bake for 9 to 12 minutes, based on your oven.

10. Remove and cool on a wire rack.

ADDITIONAL SUGGESTIONS:

You can keep these oatmeal breakfast cookies for up to three days in a covered container or freeze them for three months, reheating in the oven for a few minutes. You can substitute cranberries for raisins if you wish. You will get the same results from raisins as cranberries, in terms of digestive health and regularity.

Lunches

Lunch is often another of the much needed meals that many of us find ourselves missing on a very busy day; this is not good because in order to maintain a healthy weight as well as healthy blood sugar levels, one should never skip meals. A high protein and healthy carbohydrate rich lunch is guaranteed to help keep you going through the afternoon and avoid the vending machine at all costs. The recipes to follow are easy to prepare and can be made in advance to take on the go to work or any day out.

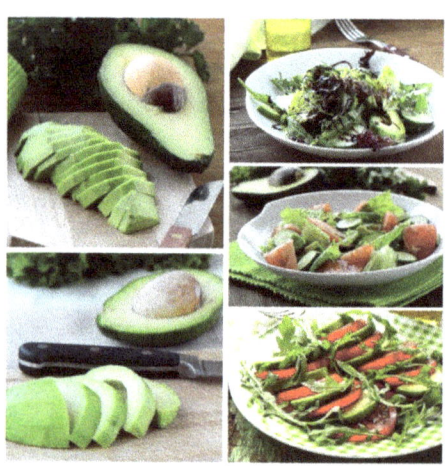

Sundried Tomato and Black Olive Frittata

Organic free range eggs are really a very versatile source of protein and can be enjoyed as a meal at any time of the day. This recipe, and the ones to follow, will show you how you can include this nutrient rich gift from nature into so many creative meal options. The sundried tomatoes not only add a wonderful flavour combination when paired with the black olives, but also provide anti-oxidants and vitamin C. The black olives add healthy essential fats.

Serves one

Preparation time: approximately 50 minutes

Ingredients:

- 2 large Organic Free Range eggs
- ¼ cup (60ml) Organic sundried tomatoes
- 1 Tablespoon (15ml) Black olives, pitted and chopped
- 1 Tablespoon (15ml) Fresh basil, chopped
- ¼ teaspoon (1.25ml) Baking powder
- Ground organic sea salt to taste
- Ground organic black pepper to taste

Instructions:

1. Preheat the oven to 350degrees (200 degrees Celsius)
2. Spray a single-serving oven proof ramekin or casserole dish with cooking spray
3. Place the sundried tomatoes, fresh chopped basil, salt, pepper and black olives into the oven proof dish, mix together
4. In a mixing bowl, crack the eggs and add the baking powder, whisk well until light and fluffy
5. Pour the whisked egg over the other ingredients that are now in the oven proof dish
6. Bake in the oven for 40-45 minutes
7. Serve with a side salad of fresh organic greens

*This frittata can be enjoyed hot or cold and will keep in the refrigerator for up to one week; it is also suitable for home freezing.

Lentil and Veggie Packed Omelet

Eggs have received a bad rep throughout the years, but truly with range free, grain feed chickens you can have healthy omelets. As long as you don't eat eggs every day you will not need to worry about cholesterol issues. Eggs are high in protein, as well as vitamin B-12. When you add in lentils and other veggies like kale, you also gain more vitamin B-12 that helps increase your metabolism and establish a healthy nervous system.

SERVES: One

PREPARATION TIME: 17 minutes, approximately

INGREDIENTS:

- 1 cup (227 grams) shredded kale
- ¾ cup (170 grams) zucchini, sliced
- ½ cup (113 grams) cherry tomatoes, halved
- 2 eggs
- 3 tablespoons (30 ml) almond milk
- ½ teaspoon (2.84 grams) oregano
- ½ cup (113 grams) lentils, cooked
- ¼ teaspoon (1.42 grams) paprika, smoked

INSTRUCTIONS:

1. Use an oil of your choice, anything you prefer as a clean cooking oil, mist the frying pan.
2. When the oil is hot, sauté the zucchini, tomatoes, and kale.
3. Sauté for 2 minutes.
4. While sautéing the veggies, whisk the eggs, milk, paprika, and oregano in a bowl.
5. Pour the egg mixture into the frying pan.
6. Mix it around with the veggies.
7. Reduce heat to medium, cook until the eggs begin to set.
8. Scatter the lentils in once the eggs start to set.
9. Cook the eggs until they are done, usually 4 to 5 minutes.
10. Flip the omelet when the top of the eggs are no longer runny.
11. Cook for an additional minute.
12. Serve.

ADDITIONAL SUGGESTIONS:

To add protein to this omelet, consider chicken. The chicken will need to be cooked before you drop it in the pan with the eggs. You can stir the chicken with the paprika and oregano, cook until no longer pink, and then add to the top of the eggs when you add in the lentils.

Zucchini Taco Boats

Zucchinis filled with free range chicken, a little cheese, veggies and spices will make for a great zucchini taco. You will have the added benefit of the zucchinis healthy properties that you do not gain from a tortilla taco shell, which makes this a cleaner way to fix one of your favorite foods. Zucchini is known to contain magnesium, vitamin A, potassium, zinc, omega-3 fatty acids, and vitamin B complex.

SERVES: Four

PREPARATION TIME: Approximately 1 hour

INGREDIENTS:

- 1 bell pepper, chopped
- 2 tablespoons (30 ml) oil
- 1 finely chopped sweet onion
- ¼ teaspoon (1.42 grams) pepper
- 1 pound (453 grams) free range chicken or turkey
- 1 tablespoon (15 ml) cumin
- ½ teaspoon (2.84 grams) paprika
- ½ teaspoon (2.84 grams) chili powder

- ½ teaspoon (2.84 grams) garlic powder
- ¼ teaspoon (1.42 grams) cayenne pepper
- 2 cups (454 grams) mixed cheeses (taco cheese mix)
- 4 zucchinis, halved, with ends cut off, and insides scooped out
- Green onions, chopped for garnish

INSTRUCTIONS:

1. Preheat oven to 400 degrees F (204 degrees C).
2. Sautee bell pepper, onion, and pepper in butter or oil for 3 to 5 minutes, or until golden brown. Use medium heat.
3. Combine the seasonings into a small bowl, mix thoroughly.
4. Add the chicken or turkey to your pan and cook for 7 to 10 minutes, or until thoroughly cooked.
5. Turn off the heat and mix in 1 ½ cup of cheese.
6. On a baking sheet, place tin foil.
7. Put the zucchini boats face up on the baking sheet.
8. Use a little oil to get the seasoning to stick.
9. Put the meat and cheese mixture into the boats.

10. Cover with aluminum foil and bake for 15 minutes.

11. Remove the foil and cook for another 10 to 15 minutes.

12. Top each boat with cheese.

13. Melt the cheese for 1 to 2 minutes.

14. Add in the green onions, plate and serve.

ADDITIONAL SUGGESTIONS:

You can use any white meat to make these taco boats. You can also adapt the seasoning ingredients to your taste, eliminating some or adding others depending on what you like.

Veggie Burgers with Avocado

Veggie burgers are a healthier way to obtain protein for your meal, than beef; especially, if you wish to lose weight. Adding in avocado helps enhance the anti-oxidants and vitamins you need to promote a healthy body. Black beans are also a great source of protein and help make this recipe a full meal.

SERVES: 4

PREPARATION TIME: approximately 20 minutes

INGREDIENTS:

- 1 package veggie burgers
- 1 avocado
- Whole wheat buns
- 1 8-ounce (28 grams) can black beans

INSTRUCTIONS:

1. In a large skillet, start cooking the veggie burgers.
2. Cook the burgers thoroughly.
3. Remove the skin and the pit of the avocado.
4. Slice the avocado into thin slices that you can place on top of your burger.

5. Cook the black beans according to the directions on the can.

6. Serve warm.

ADDITIONAL SUGGESTIONS:

You can add additional vegetables or fruit to your dinner plate for a well-rounded meal. You can also consider using onions and lettuce on top of your burger to enhance the taste.

Soba Noodles with Sesame, Kale, and Brussels Sprouts

Utilizing organic sesame seeds, kale, Brussel sprouts, and all other ingredients you can make a vegetarian dish with protein sourced from the sesame seeds and veggies. The veggies contain anti-oxidants and vitamins necessary for your health. It is a low calorie option to help you lose weight.

SERVES: Three to Four people

PREPARATION TIME: 15 minutes

INGREDIENTS:

- 8-ounce (226 grams) package of Soba Noodles
- 8 teaspoons (45.50 grams) sesame oil, divided in half
- 1 5-ounce (425 grams) package of baby kale
- 8 Brussels Sprouts
- 1 garlic clove
- 1 tablespoon (15 ml) brown rice wine vinegar
- 1 teaspoon (5.69 grams) soy sauce
- 1 tablespoon (15 ml) sesame seeds
- 2 pinches of red Chile flakes

- A handful of chives or scallions

- Sea salt to taste

INSTRUCTIONS:

1. Bring a pot of water to boil.
2. Cook the soba noodles for three minutes.
3. Drain the noodles.
4. Toss half the sesame oil in the pot with the noodles and mix.
5. While the noodles are cooking, wash and dry the veggies.
6. Prep the veggies based on type, such as removing the stems from the kale and removing the outer leaves of the Brussels sprouts.
7. In a mortar and pestle, add garlic, mash until well pounded, add in the rice vinegar, oil, and soy sauce until you create a smooth dressing.
8. Pour the dressing over the veggies and mix well.
9. Add the veggies and dressing to the noodles. The dressing will help soften the veggies, but you can also steam them with the noodles for one minute.

10. Toss the noodles, add in the sesame seeds, red Chile flakes, and pour into a serving dish.

11. Top with the chives or scallions.

12. Serve at room temperature.

ADDITIONAL SUGGESTIONS:

You can also serve this dish cold. It is best eaten the day you make it or within one day.

Roast Butternut and Goat's Cheese Frittata

This variation of the frittata recipe is very tasty and provides you with very balanced lunchtime meal. The butternut brings along essential fibre and healthy carbohydrate, while the organic goat's cheese adds some calcium to the mix; and of course we already know about the amazing health benefits of the organic free range eggs. For this recipe you would have to roast the butternut in advance; so there are two parts to this recipe.

For the roast butternut:

Preparation time: approximately 1 ½ hours

Ingredients:

- 1 large butternut, diced (it is not necessary to peel the butternut as this will retain the extra fibre and nutrients found in the skin)
- 1 large onion, peeled and chopped
- 1 Tablespoon (15ml) chopped fresh garlic
- 1 Tablespoon (15ml) chopped fresh ginger
- 1 Tablespoon (15ml) organic peach chutney
- 1 Tablespoon (15ml) mild Masala curry mix

Instructions:

1. Preheat the oven to 350 degrees, (200degrees Celsius)
2. Spray a large oven proof roasting dish with cooking spray
3. Place the butternut, onion, garlic and ginger into the roasting dish
4. Stir in the chutney and Masala mix; mix all together well
5. Roast in the oven for approximately one hour until soft and golden brown.

For the Frittata:

Serves one

Preparation time: approximately 50 minutes

Ingredients:

- 2 Organic free range eggs
- ½ Cup (125ml) roast butternut
- 1 Tablespoon (15ml) fresh coriander, finely chopped
- 2 Tablespoons (30ml) Organic Goat's Chauvin cheese, chunked
- ¼ teaspoon (1.25ml) baking powder

Instructions:

1. Spray a single serving oven proof casserole or ramekin dish with cooking spray

2. Place the roast butternut, goat's cheese and chopped coriander into the oven proof dish, mix all together

3. In a separate mixing bowl, crack the eggs and add the baking powder; whisk well until light and fluffy

4. Pour the egg mixture over the other ingredients that are in the oven proof dish

5. Bake in the oven for about 40-45 minutes

6. Serve with a side salad of fresh organic greens

*This frittata can be enjoyed hot or cold and will keep in the refrigerator for up to one week; it is also suitable for home freezing.

Fresh Hake or Cod Cakes

The many health benefits of eating freshly caught fish can be enjoyed with this recipe. Fish is very good source of protein, essential amino acids and iron; it is also very low in fat and therefore a great protein choice when watching your weight. These fish cakes are easy to prepare and are suitable for home freezing; they also make for a very convenient and easy on the go lunch.

Makes four fish cakes

Preparation time: approximately one hour.

Ingredients:

- 4 Cups (1litre) cooked hake or cod, flaked
- 2 large organic free range eggs
- 1 Tablespoon (15ml) Fresh coriander, finely chopped
- 1 teaspoon (5ml) Fresh garlic, finely chopped
- 1 teaspoon (5ml) Fresh ginger, finely chopped
- 1 teaspoon (5ml) Fresh red chili, finely chopped
- ½ teaspoon (2.5ml) Freshly ground organic black pepper
- ½ teaspoon (2.5ml) Freshly ground organic sea salt

- 1 Tablespoon (15ml) Organic Extra Virgin Olive Oil (for frying)

Instructions:

1. Place the pre-cooked hake or cod in a large mixing bowl
2. Add all the other ingredients and mix well
3. Using your hands form the mixture into four separate fish cakes
4. Place on a plate and refrigerate for approximately 30 minutes
5. Heat the Extra Virgin Olive Oil in a non-stick frying pan, on a medium to low heat.
6. Lightly fry the fish cakes until golden brown
7. Serve either hot or cold with a side salad of fresh organic greens.
8. These fish cakes would also make a really nice option for a "fish burger" when served on a 100% whole-wheat bread bun

Roast Butternut Salad with Organic Free Range Hard Boiled Eggs

This recipe provides you with a light, yet very satisfying lunch that includes all the necessities; being protein, healthy carbohydrate, healthy fats and fresh greens. As with all the lunchtime recipes in this book, this one also makes for a great on-the-go lunch.

Serves One:

Preparation time: approximately 20 minutes when you using pre-roasted butternut.

Ingredients:

- ½ Cup (125ml) Roast butternut (see recipe above)
- 2 hard-boiled organic free range eggs
- ½ Cup (125ml) Fresh coriander leaves
- ¼ Cup (60ml) Fresh Cucumber slices
- ½ cup (60ml) Fresh cherry tomatoes, halved
- 1 Tablespoon (15ml) Raw seed mix
- 1 Tablespoon (15ml) Pickled ginger

Instructions:

1. Using a large salad bowl or serving plate

2. Place the fresh coriander leaves on to the plate

3. Top the fresh coriander leaves with the cucumber slices and cherry tomatoes

4. Top the fresh coriander, cucumber slices with the roast butternut

5. Slice the hard boiled eggs into quarters and arrange them on top of the salad

6. Sprinkle over the raw seed mix and pickled ginger

7. Serve.

Chick Pea, Goat's Cheese and Organic Greens Salad

This salad has a high protein punch with the combination of chick peas and goat's cheese. The chick peas also add a little essential, fibre rich carbohydrates. What makes this salad extremely versatile is the fact that one can chose whatever type of organic greens you would prefer, or are available, at the time of making it. The dried cranberries not only add a zesty sweetness, but also bring along a dose of healthy anti-oxidants and vitamin C to the mix. This salad also makes for a great on-the-go lunchtime meal.

Serves One

Preparation time: approximately 10 minutes:

Ingredients:

- 1 Cup (250ml) Fresh organic salad greens
- ½ Cup (125ml) Chick peas, (these can be of the canned variety, just make sure they are drained and well rinsed)
- ¼ Cup (60ml) Organic Goat's cheese of your choice
- 1 Tablespoon (15ml) Raw seed mix
- 1 Tablespoon (15ml) Dried organic cranberries

Instructions:

1. Using a single serving salad bowl, assemble all the ingredients together and toss

2. Serve immediately or pack in a sealable container for and on-the-go lunch.

Organic Free Range Egg Omelette with Goat's Cheese and Free Range Smoked Trout

This omelette is high in protein, essential amino acids and Omega 3s from the smoked trout. The high nutritional value of this meal makes it a great lunchtime choice in order to avoid the mid-afternoon slump. The inclusion of baby spinach and fresh cherry tomatoes amps up the already high vitamin and mineral content of this meal; making it a rich iron source and a good choice for a recovery lunch on a day that includes high activity levels and heavy training.

Serves One

Preparation time: approximately 20 minutes

Ingredients:

- 2 Large Organic Free Range Eggs
- ¼ teaspoon (1.25ml) baking powder
- ¼ cup (60ml) Organic Goat's milk Chauvin cheese
- ½ cup (125ml) Organic free range smoked trout
- ¼ cup (60ml) Organic fresh baby spinach
- ¼ cup (60ml) Organic fresh cherry tomatoes, halved

Instructions:

1. Crack the eggs into a mixing bowl, and the baking powder and whisk well until light and fluffy
2. Spray a non-stick frying pan with cooking spray and place it on the stove top at a medium heat
3. Pour the beaten eggs into the frying pan and allow to cook
4. When the omelette begins to lift around the edges, gently turn it over to cook on the other side.
5. Once the omelette is completely cooked, place it on a large dinner plate
6. Cover half of the omelette with the baby spinach leaves
7. Top the baby spinach leaves with the cherry tomatoes
8. Top the baby spinach and cherry tomatoes with the free range smoked trout
9. Place the Goat's milk Chauvin cheese on top of the free range smoked trout
10. Fold the omelette over and serve with whole grain bread of your choice, (for example; organic 100% rye bread)

Quinoa Salad with Seared Free-Range Tuna

Fresh tuna is high in essential amino acids and Omega 3s, it is also a very great source of protein. Quinoa provides this meal with a wholesome, high fibre carbohydrate that is also high in protein. This salad is a great lunchtime option because it is well balanced and satisfying; it is guaranteed to keep your blood sugar levels stable throughout the afternoon.

Serves One

Preparation time: approximately 20 minutes

Ingredients:

- ½ Cup (125ml) Cooked quinoa
- 1 medium-sized fresh free-range tuna steak
- 1 Tablespoon (15ml) Organic Extra virgin Olive Oil
- 1 Tablespoon (15ml) Freshly ground organic black pepper
- 1 Tablespoon (15ml) Fresh organic lime juice
- 1 Cup (250ml) Fresh organic baby spinach
- ½ Cup (125ml) Fresh organic cherry tomatoes, halved
- ½ of a medium-sized avocado, sliced
- 1 Tablespoon (15ml) Raw sesame seeds

- 1 Tablespoon (15ml) Pickled ginger

Instructions:

1. Cover the base of a non-stick frying pan with the extra virgin olive oil
2. Place the pan on the stove top on a high heat
3. Cover the tuna steak on both sides with the freshly ground black pepper
4. Sear the tuna on both sides in the hot olive oil coated pan
5. Once the tuna is seared and "crispy" on both sides, remove it from the heat and place on a plate
6. In a single serving salad bowl, place the cooked quinoa and top it with the organic fresh baby spinach and cherry tomatoes
7. Slice the seared tuna steak into as many slices as desired
8. Arrange the tuna steak slices over the other ingredients that are already in salad bowl
9. Arrange the avocado slices over the seared tuna
10. Sprinkle over the raw sesame seeds and the pickled ginger

11. Just before serving, drizzle the organic fresh lime juice over the entire salad.

Healthy Snacks

One of the keys to achieving and maintaining a healthy weight is eat small meals throughout the day, therefore the inclusion of a healthy snack in between breakfast and lunch, and then again in between lunch and dinner is actually a necessity to living a healthy lifestyle. This section of the book provide you with recipes and creative ideas for healthy, blood sugar sustaining snacks that are easy to prepare and won't have you reaching for sweets or fried potato chips.

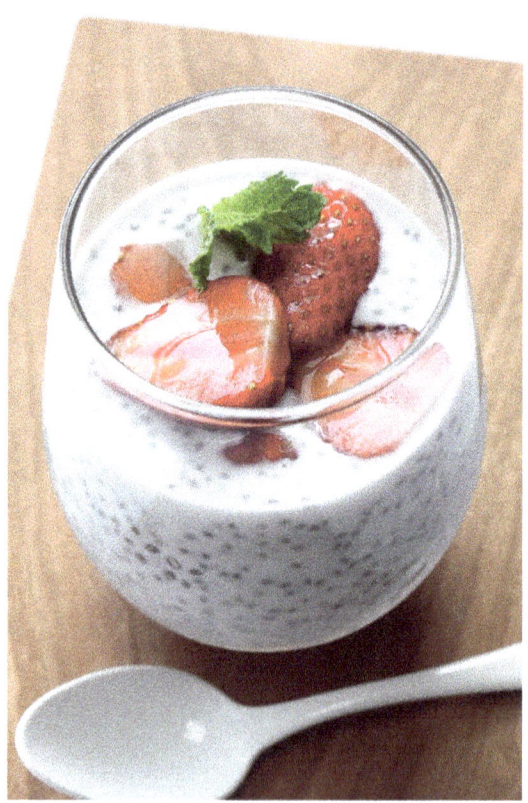

Organic Granny Smith Apple Slices with Fresh Ginger and Chopped Pecan Nuts

Apples have a low glycaemic index, making them a very great snack choice when looking to stave off hunger in a healthy way. Fresh ginger is high in anti-inflammatory and immune boosting properties, and the pecan nuts add a healthy crunch as well as healthy fats and extra essential minerals. By drizzling over the apple cider vinegar you are adding all the health benefits that it processes, including its ability to stabilise and balance the body's pH levels as well as boost metabolism.

Serves One

Preparation time: approximately 10 minutes:

Ingredients:

- 1 medium sized Organic Granny Smith apple, sliced
- 1 teaspoon (5ml) freshly grated ginger
- 1 teaspoon (5ml) ground mixed baking spice
- 1 Tablespoon (15ml) raw pecan nuts, chopped
- 1 teaspoon (5ml) Organic apple cider vinegar

Instructions:

1. Place the Organic Granny Smith apple slices in a small bowl

2. Sprinkle the chopped raw pecan nuts over the apple slices

3. Sprinkle the freshly chopped ginger and mixed baking spice over the apple slices and pecan nuts

4. Lastly, drizzle with the organic apple cider vinegar

5. You can either serve immediately or place in an airtight container to take on the go.

Organic Red Apple Slices with Organic Peanut Butter and Dried Cranberries

The combination of apple and peanut butter makes a great snack due to its fantastic balance of healthy carbohydrate and fat. The addition of the dried cranberries to this mix gives it an extra punch of anti-oxidants and healthy blood sugar sustaining carbohydrates, keeping your metabolism fired up.

Serves One

Preparation time: approximately 10 minutes

Ingredients:

- 1 medium sized organic red apple, sliced
- 1 Tablespoon (15ml) organic peanut butter
- 1 teaspoon (5ml) ground baking spice mix
- 1 Tablespoon (15ml) dried cranberries

Instructions:

1. Place the apple slices in a small bowl or container
2. Add the peanut butter
3. Sprinkle the ground mixed spice over the apple and peanut butter

4. Lastly sprinkle over the dried cranberries

5. Mix to make sure that all ingredients are covered in peanut butter

6. Serve immediately or pack in an airtight container to take on the go.

Organic Goat's Cheese with Fresh Organic Crudités

The combination of healthy protein and high fibre fresh crudités in this healthy snack recipe are bound to help keep your energy levels up in a tasty and satisfying way. The choice of crudités is completely up to you, making this snack idea easy to adapt to your personal tastes and to availability of organic fresh produce. The addition of the raw seed mix adds a healthy crunch as well as essential fats.

Serves One

Preparation time: approximately 10 minutes

Ingredients:

- 1 Cup (250ml) assorted fresh organic crudités of your choice (for example; snow peas; carrot sticks, baby corn, cucumber sticks, baby cherry tomatoes, fresh green beans, etc.)

- 1 Cup (250ml) Organic goat's cheese of your choice

- 1 Tablespoon (15ml) Raw seed mix

- Freshly ground organic black pepper and sea salt to taste

Instructions:

1. Place all the crudités on a serving plate, season with the freshly ground black pepper and sea salt

2. In a separate bowl place the organic goat's cheese and sprinkle over the raw seed mix

3. Serve immediately or place in sealable containers to take on the go

Fresh Organic Berries with Organic Goat's Milk Yogurt and Raw Almonds

Fresh berries are a rich source of anti-oxidants, vitamins and minerals. The goat's milk yogurt provides a healthy dose of calcium and amino acids. The addition of raw almonds brings along some healthy fats and extra essential vitamins and minerals. The raw cocoa powder adds extra anti-oxidants and a very healthy chocolatey taste. Raw honey provides a little healthy sweetness.

Serves One

Preparation time: approximately 10 minutes

Ingredients:

- 1 Cup (250ml) Mixed fresh organic berries (for example; black berries, cherries, blueberries, goose berries and strawberries)
- 1 Cup (250ml) Plan organic goat's milk yogurt
- 1 teaspoon (5ml) Raw cocoa powder
- 1 Tablespoon (15ml) Raw almonds, chopped
- 1 Tablespoon (15ml) Raw organic honey

Instructions:

1. Place the berry mix into a small serving bowl

2. Top the berries with the organic goat's milk yogurt

3. Sprinkle the raw cocoa powder over the goat's milk yogurt

4. Sprinkle the chopped raw almonds over the berries and goat's milk yogurt

5. Lastly, drizzle the raw organic honey over all the other ingredients

6. Serve immediately or place in an airtight container to take on the go.

Fresh Organic Avocado Guacamole with Fresh Organic Crudités

Fresh avocados are incredibly healthy since they are high in heart-healthy fats and essential vitamins and minerals such as folic acid and potassium. The wholesome and nutritious qualities that avocados possess make them a very satisfying snack choice.

Serves One

Preparation time: approximately 10 minutes

Ingredients:

- ½ a ripe avocado, peeled, pitted and cut into chunks
- 1 teaspoon (5ml) Organic Balsamic vinegar
- Freshly ground organic black pepper and sea salt to taste
- ¼ cup (60ml) Organic goat's milk Chauvin cheese
- 1 cup (250ml) assorted fresh organic crudités of your choice (for example; snow peas; carrot sticks, baby corn, cucumber sticks, baby cherry tomatoes, fresh green beans, etc.)

Instructions:

1. Place the avocado chunks into a small bowl

2. Add the organic Balsamic vinegar

3. Add the freshly ground organic black pepper and sea salt

4. Add the organic goat's milk Chauvin cheese

5. Mix all the ingredients together with a fork until you have a guacamole texture

6. Place the crudités on a serving plate with the bowl of guacamole on the side as a dip for the crudités

Dinners

A healthy, wholesome dinner is essential for achieving and maintaining a healthy weight and for keeping your metabolism fired up throughout the long fast of sleeping. A healthy dinner needs to consist of a good balance of healthy protein, carbohydrate and fats in order to ensure that you are ending your day on the healthiest note possible. The dinner recipes in this section are easy to prepare, and will ensure that you won't wake in the middle of the night hungry, even though they are light enough so as not to cause digestive discomfort while sleeping. As an added bonus, most of the recipes to follow make for great leftovers that can be packed for on-the-go lunches for the following day; they are also suitable for home freezing making them even more versatile.

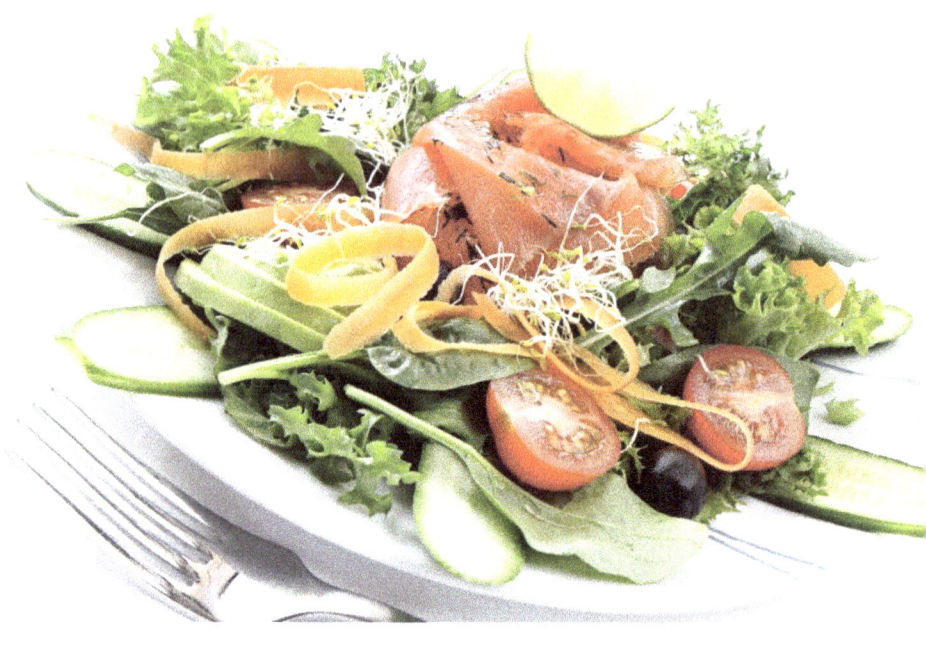

Fresh Free Range Salmon Curry with Coconut Milk, Roast Butternut and Brown Rice

Fresh salmon is very high in essential Omega 3s and amino acids; it is very high in protein, making this recipe an excellent dinner choice when you are wanting to achieve a healthy, strong immune system through your dietary choices. The addition of roast butternut and brown rice adds essential fibre and slow releasing carbohydrates to fill you up and stave off hunger throughout the night.

Serves One

Preparation time: approximately 40 minutes, if using pre-roasted butternut

Ingredients:

- 1 medium sized fresh free range salmon steak, cut into chunks
- ½ Cup (125ml) Roast butternut (see recipe in Lunch section of this book)
- ½ Cup (125ml) Cooked brown rice
- ½ Cup (125ml) Coconut milk
- 1 Tablespoon (15ml) Desiccated coconut

Instructions:

1. Spray a single serving oven proof dish (preferably one with a lid) with cooking spray

2. Place the cooked brown rice in the bottom of the oven proof dish

3. Place the roast butternut on top of the brown rice

4. Place the fresh salmon chunks on top of the butternut

5. Pour the coconut milk over all the ingredients

6. Cover the dish with its lid and bake in the oven for 40 minutes (if your dish does not have a lid, you can cover it with foil)

7. Once baked, sprinkle over the desiccated coconut and serve

Baked Fresh Free Range Hake or Cod with Roast Vegetables and Quinoa

This recipe provides a light, yet hearty and wholesome dinner. The roast vegetables can be made in advance and used as a side dish to any meal; they can also be used as a base for other recipes.

For the roast vegetables:

Preparation time: approximately one hour

Preheat the oven to 350 degrees (200 degrees Celsius)

Ingredients:

- 1 Cup (250ml) Assorted fresh organic peppers (red, green and orange)
- 1 Cup (250ml) Fresh organic cherry tomatoes, halved
- 1 Cup (250ml) Sundried tomatoes
- 1 Cup (250ml) Fresh organic zucchini, sliced
- 1 large red onion, finely chopped
- 1 Tablespoon (15ml) fresh garlic, finely chopped
- 1 Cup (250ml) Fresh basil, finely chopped
- Freshly ground organic black pepper and sea salt to taste

- 1 Tablespoon (15ml) Organic Extra virgin olive oil

Instructions:

1. Spray a large baking or roasting pan with cooking spray
2. Place all the ingredients into the baking or roasting pan
3. Cover the ingredients with the olive oil, making sure they are all well coated
4. Roast in the oven for 50 minutes
5. After 50 minutes, turn the oven off and allow the vegetables to cool in the oven.

For the fish dish:

Serves One

Preparation time: approximately 35 minutes

Ingredients:

- 1 medium sized piece of fresh free range hake or cod
- Freshly ground organic black pepper and sea salt to taste
- 1 Tablespoon (15ml) fresh organic lemon juice
- ½ Cup (125ml) cooked quinoa
- 1 Cup (250ml) roast vegetables

- ½ of a ripe avocado, sliced

Instructions:

Preheat the oven to 350 degrees (200 degrees Celsius)

1. Spray a oven proof dish with cooking spray
2. Place the hake or cod in the oven proof dish and sprinkle with the freshly ground black pepper and sea salt
3. Drizzle with the lemon juice
4. Bake in the oven for 35 minutes
5. Place the quinoa and roast vegetables on a serving plate
6. Once the hake or cod is cooked, place it on the serving plate with the quinoa and roast vegetables, top the fish with the sliced avocado and serve

Whole Wheat Pasta Bake with Roast Vegetables, Black Olives and Goat's Milk Cheese

Whole wheat pasta is a great alternative to the highly refined white variety, and is a better choice due to its high fibre content which gives it a much lower glycaemic index making it a wonderful dinner option to stave off night time hunger. The roast vegetables add to the high fibre content of this recipe and the black olives bring along the healthy fats; the goat's milk cheese adds protein to make this a well-balanced meal.

Serve One

Preparation time: approximately 35 minutes, if using pre-cooked roast vegetables

Ingredients:

- ½ Cup (125ml) cooked whole wheat past
- 1 Cup (250ml) roast vegetables (see recipe above)
- 1 Tablespoon (15ml) Black olives, pitted and sliced
- ¼ Cup (60ml) Organic goat's milk Chauvin cheese

Instructions:

Prcheat the oven to 350 degrees (200 degrees Celsius)

1. Spay a single serving oven proof dish (preferably one with a lid) with cooking spray

2. Place the cooked whole wheat pasta in the bottom of the oven proof dish

3. Place the roast vegetables on top of the cooked pasta

4. Place the organic goat's milk Chauvin cheese on top of the roast vegetables

5. Sprinkle the sliced black olives over the goat's milk Chauvin cheese

6. Cover with the lid (or foil if your dish doesn't have a lid) and bake for 25 minutes, serve immediately

Roast Vegetable and Black Olive Patties

This recipe provides a great option for a healthy vegetarian burger, by using the blended chick peas as a binding agent, along with the organic free range egg; you are adding essential protein to the already fibre-rich roast vegetables. These patties can be made in advance and stored in the freezer for convenience.

Makes four patties

Preparation time: approximately one hour, if using pre-cooked roast veg

Ingredients:

- 2 Cups (500ml) Roast vegetables (see recipe above)
- 2 large organic free range eggs, beaten
- 2 cups (500ml) Chick peas, the canned variety is easiest but make sure they are drained and well rinsed
- ¼ Cup (60ml) Tahini
- ¼ Cup (60ml) Black olives, pitted and sliced
- 1 tablespoon (15ml) Organic Extra Virgin olive oil
- ½ of a ripe avocado

Instructions:

1. Place the chick peas and Tahini into a food processor and blitz into a smooth paste

2. Place the roast veg, organic free range eggs and black olives into a mixing bowl

3. Mix all the ingredients together and then form into four patties

4. Place the patties on a plate and refrigerate for about 30 minutes

5. After the patties have been in the refrigerator for 30 minutes, place the extra virgin olive oil into a non-stick pan and place it on the stove top at a medium heat

6. Cook the patties in the pan until golden brown on either side.

7. Serve on a whole wheat bread bun with the ripe avocado and a side salad of fresh organic greens.

Vegetarian Chili with Brown Rice and Black Olives

This recipe is a hearty, wholesome carbohydrate and protein rich meal that provides a healthy meat free alternative to the traditional chili recipe. The red kidney beans are packed with fibre and high in protein and together with the brown rice this combination will fill you up without causing any discomfort to the digestive system, it will also keep you full all night.

Serves Four

Preparation time: approximately one hour

Ingredients:

- 2 Cups (500ml) cooked brown rice

- 2 Cups (500ml) red kidney beans, the canned variety will be easiest just make sure that they are drained and well rinsed

- 1 Cup (250ml) chopped fresh organic tomatoes

- 1 medium sized red onion, finely chopped

- 1 Tablespoon (15ml) fresh garlic, finely chopped

- 1 Tablespoon (15ml) fresh red chillies, finely chopped

- ¼ Cup (60ml) Organic tomato paste

- Freshly ground organic black pepper and sea salt to taste
- 1 teaspoon (5ml) chilli powder
- 1 Tablespoon (15ml) Organic extra virgin olive oil
- 1 Cup (250ml) black olives, pitted and sliced

Instructions:

1. Heat the extra virgin olive oil in a saucepan
2. Lightly fry the onion, garlic and chili
3. Add the chopped organic tomatoes, black olives, tomato paste and red kidney beans
4. Add the chili powder, black pepper and sea salt
5. Stir all together and allow to simmer for approximately 30-40 minutes, until the red kidney beans are soft
6. Using four separate serving bowls, place ½ cup (125ml) of the cooked brown rice into each bowl
7. Top each bowl of rice with 1 cup (250ml) of the cooked vegetarian chili and serve hot
8. This vegetarian chili is very suitable for home freezing.

Fresh Whole Free Range Trout with Fresh Organic Greens

Fresh trout is another fish option that is packed with healthy Omega 3s and high in protein. Cooking the freshly caught free range fish whole provides a fresh approach. This recipe is inspired by the flavours of Thailand and proves how healthy eating doesn't have to be boring or tasteless.

Serves two

Preparation time: approximately one hour

Ingredients:

- 1 whole fresh free range trout, gutted and cleaned
- ¼ cup (60ml) Fresh ginger, finely chopped
- 2 Tablespoons (30ml) Fresh garlic, finely chopped
- 1 Tablespoon (15ml) Fresh red chili, finely chopped
- ¼ Cup (60ml) Fresh organic lime juice
- 2 Tablespoons (30ml) Lime zest
- 2 Tablespoons (30ml) Desiccated coconut

Instructions:

Preheat the oven to 350 degrees (200 degrees Celsius)

1. Spray and oven proof baking dish or tray with cooking spray
2. Place the whole trout on the bottom of the baking dish or tray
3. Cover the fish with the garlic, chilli, ginger, lime zest and desiccated coconut
4. Drizzle over the fresh lime juice
5. Bake in the oven for 35-40 minutes until the skin of the fish is crispy
6. Serve with a side salad of fresh organic greens of your choice
7. This meal can also be served with cooked brown rice to add a little high fibre healthy carbohydrate

Vegetarian Lasagne with Organic Goat's Cheese Topping

This lasagne uses whole wheat lasagne sheets, making it a healthier alternative to the normal highly refined white pasta sheets. Furthermore, this lasagne is not made with the creamy béchamel sauce that the traditional variety is made with, making it lower in unhealthy fats and lighter on the digestive system. This lasagne is very suitable for home freezing and can be made in advance in these single serving portions for convenience.

Serves One

Preparation time: approximately one hour

Ingredients:

- Whole wheat lasagne sheets
- 2 Cups (500ml) roast vegetables (see recipe above)
- ¼ Cup (60ml) black olives, pitted and sliced
- ¼ Cup (60ml) organic goat's milk cheese, grated

Instructions:

Preheat the oven to 350 degrees (200 degrees Celsius)

- Spray a single serving oven proof dish or ramekin with cooking spray

- Place a layer of the lasagne sheets on the bottom off the dish
- Place a layer of the roast vegetables on top of the lasagne sheets
- Place a layer of the black olives over the roast vegetables
- Begin again with the lasagne sheets and continue to layer as above until the dish is full
- Sprinkle the grated goat's cheese over the top of the lasagne
- Bake in the oven for approximately 40-45 minutes
- Serve with a side salad of fresh organic greens.

Chick Pea and Sweet Potato Curry with Quinoa

This high protein, high fibre curry dish is a great dinner option on a cold winter night. It's very filling and will keep you full all night. This recipe is another of those that is very suitable for home freezing and can be made in advance in single servings to freeze for later convenience.

Serves Four

Preparation time: approximately one and a half hours

Ingredients:

- 2 Cups (500ml) Cooked quinoa
- 2 Cups (500ml) Sweet potato , cubed
- 2 Cups (500ml) Chick peas
- 1 Tablespoon (15ml) Fresh garlic, finely chopped
- 1 Tablespoon (15ml) Fresh ginger, finely chopped
- 1 Tablespoon (15ml) Fresh red chilli, finely chopped
- 1 Tablespoon (15ml) Mild masala curry mix
- 1 teaspoon (5ml) cumin seeds
- 1 teaspoon (5ml) ground coriander

- 2 Cups (500ml) Coconut milk
- 1 large onion, finely chopped
- 1 Tablespoon (15ml) Organic extra virgin olive oil

Instructions:

1. Heat the olive oil in a saucepan
2. Fry the onion, garlic, chilli and ginger until soft
3. Add the chick peas and sweet potato
4. Add the coconut milk
5. Bring to a simmer and allow to cook for about 40 minutes.
6. Using four separate serving bowls, place ½ cup (125ml) of the cooked quinoa in each bowl
7. Place 1 Cup (250ml) of the chick pea and sweet potato curry into each bowl
8. Serve hot

Chicken with Brussels Sprouts and Mustard Sauce

The preparation and cooking time of this recipe may seem like a long time, but it is in fact one of the best go-to recipes for you to use during your busy week. You can prepare this meal in a slow cooker to ensure it is cooking during the day or you can simply make it when you get home. Brussels sprouts are known to contain healthy vitamins, while the free range chicken will keep it a clean meal.

SERVES: Four (serving size: 1 half chicken breast, 2/3 cup Brussels sprouts and 2 tablespoons sauce)

PREPARATION TIME: Approximately 40 minutes

INGREDIENTS:

- 2 tablespoons (30 ml) olive oil, divided
- 3/8 teaspoon (2.13 grams) salt, divided
- ¼ teaspoon (1.42 grams) freshly ground black pepper
- 4 6-ounce (170 grams) boneless, halve chicken breasts
- ¾ cup (180 ml) fat-free, low-sodium chicken broth, divided
- 2 tablespoons (30 ml) unfiltered apple cider
- 2 tablespoons (30 ml) whole grain Dijon mustard
- 1 tablespoon (15 ml) fresh flat-leaf parsley chopped
- 2 tablespoons (30 ml) butter, divided (you can use coconut oil instead)

- 12 ounces (340 grams) Brussels sprouts, halved and trimmed

INSTRUCTIONS:

1. Preheat oven to 450 degrees
2. Using a large ovenproof skillet, heat over high heat
3. Scatter chicken with ¼ teaspoon salt and pepper; then add to pan
4. Cook 3 minutes or until lightly browned
5. Turn chicken; place the pan in the oven
6. Bake in a 450-degree oven for approximately 9 minutes or until done
7. Keep the chicken warm after removing from pan
8. Heat the pan over medium-high heat; add ½ cup broth and cider
9. Bring to a boil while scraping the browned bits from sides and bottom of pan
10. Lower the heat to medium-low and simmer for 4 minutes. The mixture should thicken
11. With a whisk, add mustard, 1 tablespoon butter and parsley
12. Add 1 tablespoon of oil along with 1 tablespoon of butter in a large non- stick frying pan over medium-high heat
13. Add Brussels sprouts; sauté about two minutes or until light brown
14. Add 1/8 teaspoon salt and ¼ cup broth to pan

15. Cover and cook approximately 4 minutes or till tender crisp
16. Serve Brussels sprouts with chicken and sauce

ADDITIONAL SUGGESTIONS:

Consider pairing this meal with oven-roasted rosemary potatoes. You may also use different spices if you prefer. Simply use coconut oil to keep the potatoes clean and healthier than butter or olive oil.

Lemony Chicken Kebabs with Tomato Salad

Lemon is a known containing calcium, citric acid, and magnesium. The free range chicken you will use for this recipe keeps it healthy and adds protein to your meal. With the various spices you will use for the tomato salad and chicken kebabs, you will enhance your digestion, metabolism speed, and lose weight.

SERVES: Four

PREPARATION TIME: Approximately 2 hours, 25 minutes

INGREDIENTS:

- Divide, 3 tablespoons (45 ml) fresh squeezed lemon juice
- 1 ½ teaspoons (8.53 grams) dried oregano, divided
- 1 tablespoon (15 ml) garlic, minced and divided
- ¾ teaspoon (4.27 grams) kosher salt, divided
- 3 tablespoons (45 ml) extra-virgin olive oil, divided
- ¾ teaspoon (4.27 grams) freshly ground black pepper, divided
- 4 (6 ounce or 170 grams) chicken breast halves, boneless, cut into 1 ½ inch cubes
- 1 cup (240 ml) chopped cherry tomatoes
- 2 cups (480 ml) fresh parsley leaves

INSTRUCTIONS:

1. Combine 2 teaspoons garlic, 2 tablespoons lemon juice, ½ teaspoon salt, ½ teaspoon pepper and 1 teaspoon oregano
2. Add to mixture 1 tablespoon oil and stir with a whisk.
3. Put the chicken into the marinade and stir. Marinate for 2 hours in the refrigerator, covered.
4. Remove chicken from the mixture and discard the marinade.
5. Place the chicken on skewers. Use 4, 10 inch skewers.
6. Preheat a grill pan over high heat.
7. Add the skewers, turn them often; cook for 6 minutes or until done.
8. The remaining 1 tablespoon lemon juice, ½ teaspoon oregano, 1 teaspoon garlic, 1/4 teaspoon salt and pepper are combined in a medium bowl.
9. Slowly add the final 2 tablespoons of oil, whisk until well blended.
10. Combine parsley and tomatoes with the contents of a bowl and toss to coat.
11. Place salad on plate and top with skewers.

ADDITIONAL SUGGESTIONS:

If you are going to be short of time, the marinating time can be cut in half. The flavors will still mingle and the lemony goodness will shine through.

Mediterranean Stuffed Chicken Breasts

A Mediterranean diet is one of the healthiest on the planet. This simple to prepare dish is perfect for a quick weeknight supper, yet fancy enough for guests. The free range chicken keeps this as a healthy recipe that you can use each week. With different veggies on the side, you can always add to the vitamins you receive.

SERVES: Eight (serving: one half stuffed chicken breast)

PREPARATION TIME: Approximately 45 minutes

INGREDIENTS:

- 8 (6 ounce or 170 grams) boneless, skinless chicken breasts
- 1 large bell pepper
- 1 tablespoon (15 ml) fresh basil, minced
- ¼ cup (60 ml) feta cheese, crumbled
- 2 tablespoons (30 ml) finely chopped Kalamata olives, pitted

INSTRUCTIONS:

1. Preheat broiler or grill.
2. Once the bell pepper is sliced in half lengthwise, remove and discard membranes and seeds.
3. Place pepper strips on a foil lined baking sheet, with skin side up. Flatten with the heal of your hand.

4. Broil or grill for 15 minutes or until blackened to desired color.
5. Remove from baking sheet and place in a zippered plastic bag.
6. Let the bell pepper rest for 15 minutes.
7. Peel and chop into fine pieces.
8. Broiler or grill should be on medium-high heat.
9. Mix bell pepper, olives, cheese, and basil together.
10. With a knife, cut a horizontal slit in each chicken breast at the thickest portion. This will form a pocket for the mixture.
11. Insert 2 tablespoons of the bell pepper mixture in the horizontal slit.
12. Close the slit with a wooden toothpick.
13. Take a ¼ teaspoon of salt and pepper, each and sprinkle on top the of the chicken breasts.
14. Coat grill with a cooking spray.
15. Each side is grilled for 6 minutes or until done.
16. Remove from broiler or grill, cover with foil loosely.
17. Let the finished chicken breasts rest for 10 minutes.

ADDITIONAL SUGGESTIONS:

If there is a chill in the air, which makes grilling impossible a broiler can be used just as effectively. You will still enjoy a healthy, clean meal.

Shrimp and Avocado Rolls

To keep this recipe clean and for weight loss, you are going to turn it into a summer roll versus a spring roll. Instead of frying the roll, you make the rolls with fresh ingredients and avoid frying them. You don't have to use shrimp if you are allergic to shrimp or do not like the taste. Any white meat or fish can be used in these rolls.

SERVES: One

PREPARATION TIME: Approximately 20 minutes

INGREDIENTS:

- Red leaf lettuce, chopped
- 9 large shrimp
- 2 medium carrots, julienned
- 1 cup (227 grams) red cabbage, finely chopped
- 1 avocado
- 1 medium cucumber, julienned
- 1 tablespoon (15 ml) rice vinegar
- A pinch of finely chopped fresh basil
- A pinch of finely chopped fresh cilantro

- Spring roll wrappers

INSTRUCTIONS:

1. Fill a pie plate with hot water, just enough to submerge one spring roll wrapper at a time.
2. Soak each wrapper for 10 to 30 minutes, use four to six wrappers.
3. Lay the wrapper on parchment paper.
4. Place 3 shrimp halves in each wrapper. You want to arrange the shrimp to be from tip to tip of the wrapper versus leaving the wrapper square to your body.
5. Arrange the veggies along the side of the shrimp, so there is about an inch of wrapper on each side of the veggies.
6. Fold the corner of the wrapper, closest to your body, up. Fold in each side tip of the wrapper in over the veggie/shrimp mixture. Continue to roll the wrapper until the fourth corner lays over the top of the roll.
7. Set aside, until all of the wrappers have been rolled.
8. Cut the wrappers in half.
9. Arrange on a plate and serve with a dipping sauce of your choice.

ADDITIONAL SUGGESTIONS:

You will need to add steps if you do not have cooked shrimp. Make sure the shrimp or any protein added to the wrappers is thoroughly cooked and cooled before you put the ingredients in the wrappers. Most spring roll wrappers come with instructions on how to wrap the rolls, if you need them. You can also purchase gluten free, vegan wrappers for a healthier summer roll.

Thai Chopped Salad with Curry Coconut Dressing

You can never go wrong with a salad, with Thai spices. For centuries, Asian and Indian spices have been known for their health properties. A combination of Thai spices and curry will help you lose weight, as well as feel more energetic. Since this is a salad it is fairly easy to make and transport. It is one of the recipes that will make a great lunch, without making you tired on the job after your meal. You certainly won't be reaching for more coffee because you feel stuffed and fatigued.

SERVES: One

PREPARATION TIME: 20 minutes

INGREDIENTS:

- ¼ cup (60 ml) creamy peanut butter
- 1 cup (240) coconut milk
- 1 tablespoon (15 ml) yellow curry powder
- 1 lime, juice it, keep the juice
- 1 garlic clove
- 1 teaspoon (5.69 grams) Sriracha
- 3 cups (681 grams) kale, chopped

- 1 red bell pepper, finely chopped
- 2 cups (454 grams) Napa cabbage, finely chopped
- 1 cup (227 grams) carrots, shredded
- ½ cup (113 grams) peanuts, chopped
- 1 cup (227 grams) mango, chopped
- ½ cup (113 grams) cilantro, fresh and chopped

INSTRUCTIONS:

1. From the peanut butter to the Sriracha place in a blender.
2. Mix on high speed, until the mixture is smooth.
3. Place the mixture in a pot and bring it to a boil.
4. Reduce the heat and let the mixture thicken. It should take 10 minutes.
5. Set the mixture aside to cool.
6. Once you have chopped the veggies, place in a bowl.
7. Top with the dressing

ADDITIONAL SUGGESTIONS:

This can be a vegetarian meal or one with protein. Simply add a little prep time and a half pound of turkey, chicken, or fish. You will want to cook the meat thoroughly, let it cool, and place on top of your salad before you add the dressing. If you are taking this as your lunch, keep the dressing on the side, until you are ready to eat.

Goodbye and Good Natural Health

We hope you have enjoyed this book on clean eating and that you will start using the recipes as part of your weight loss and health arsenal, or vitality boosting routines.

We have a series of ebooks on various Natural Health Remedies and how to enhance your life through Mindful practices. Our wish for you is to live happily and healthily in the present moment and to enjoy every moment of your life. You are always welcome to get in touch with us, and we look forward to helping you.

For more information & resources, please visit:

www.HolisticWellnessBooks.com

Until next time

Be Beautiful, Be Healthy, Be Happy…

Finally, if you have a second, please review this book on Amazon.

Even one sentence review will do and I'd be really happy to hear from you!

I hope you will enjoy your clean eating journey

I hope to "see" you in my next book.

Love,

Cassia Albinson

Free eBook + Free Wellness Newsletter

We have a free, complimentary eBook for you.

It's waiting for you at:

www.YourWellnessBooks.com/newsletter

Problems with your download?

Email us at: info@yourwellnessbooks.com

More Books Written by Cassia

Available in Your Local Amazon Store

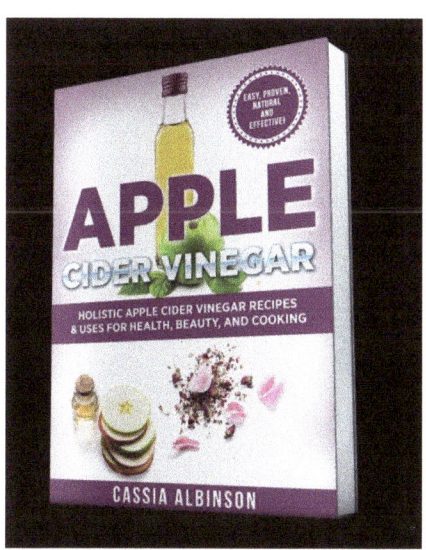

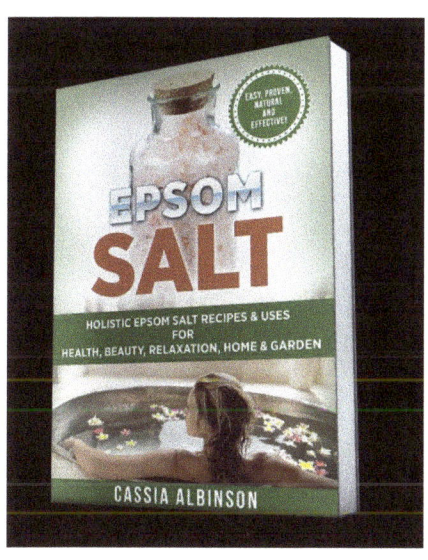

www.ingramcontent.com/pod-product-compliance
Lightning Source LLC
Chambersburg PA
CBHW042117100526
44587CB00025B/4085